The Vibrant Snack and I Guide

CW00661353

Enjoy Your Breaks with Cheap and Healthy Snacks to _
Weight

Bella Francis

contained within this document, including, but not limited to, —
errors, omissions, or inaccuracies.

Table of contents

Chocolate Crunch Bars

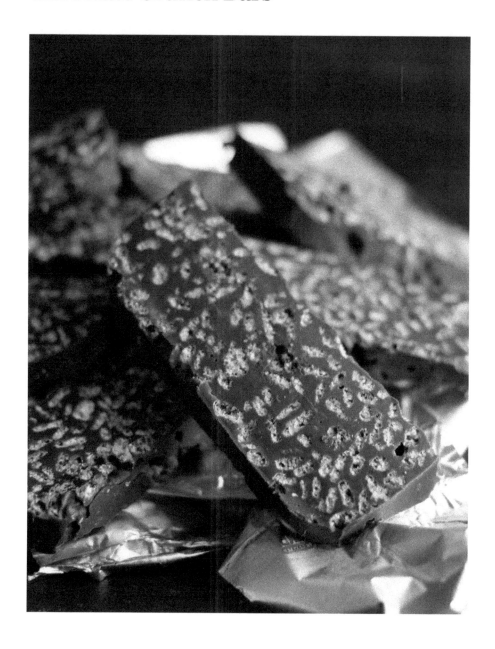

Preparation Time: 5 minutes

Cooking Time: 5 minutes

Servings: 4

Ingredients :

• 1 1/2 cups sugar-free chocolate chips

• 1 cup almond butter

• Stevia to taste

• 1/4 cup coconut oil

• 3 cups pecans , chopped

Directions:

1. Layer an 8-inch baking pan with parchment paper.

2. Mix chocolate chips with butter, coconut oil, and sweetener in a bowl.

3. Melt it by heating in a microwave for 2 to 3 minutes until well mixed.

4. Stir in nuts and seeds. Mix gently.

5. Pour this batter carefully into the baking pan and spread evenly.

6. Refrigerate for 20 minutes.

7. Slice and serve.

Nutrition:

Calories 316

Total Fat 30.9 g

Saturated Fat 8.1 g

Cholesterol 0 mg

Total Carbs 8.3 g

Sugar 1.8 g

Fiber 3.8 g

Sodium 8 mg

Protein 6.4 g

Homemade Protein Bar

Preparation Time: 5 minutes

Cooking Time: 10 minutes

Servings: 4

Ingredients :

- 1 cup nut butter
- 4 tablespoons coconut oil
- 2 scoops vanilla protein
- Stevia, to taste
- ½ teaspoon sea salt
- Optional Ingredients
- 1 teaspoon cinnamon

Directions:

1. Mix coconut oil with butter, protein, stevia, and salt in a dish.

2. Stir in cinnamon and chocolate chip.

3. Press the mixture firmly and freeze until firm.

4. Cut the crust into small bars.

5. Serve and enjoy.

Nutrition:

Calories 179

Total Fat 15.7 g

Saturated Fat 8 g

Cholesterol 0 mg

Total Carbs 4.8 g

Sugar 3.6 g

Fiber 0.8 g

Sodium 43 mg

Protein 5.6 g

Shortbread Cookies

Preparation Time: 10 minutes

Cooking Time: 70 minutes

Servings: 6

Ingredients :

- 2 1/2 cups almond flour

- 6 tablespoons nut butter

- 1/2 cup erythritol

- 1 teaspoon vanilla essence

Directions:

1. Preheat your oven to 350 degrees F.

2. Layer a cookie sheet with parchment paper.

3. Beat butter with erythritol until fluffy.

4. Stir in vanilla essence and almond flour. Mix well until becomes crumbly.

5. Spoon out a tablespoon of cookie dough onto the cookie sheet.

6. Add more dough to make as many cookies.

7. Bake for 15 minutes until brown.

8. Serve.

Nutrition:

Calories 288

Total Fat 25.3 g

Saturated Fat 6.7 g

Cholesterol 23 mg

Total Carbs 9.6 g

Sugar 0.1 g

Fiber 3.8 g

Sodium 74 mg

Potassium 3 mg

Protein 7.6 g

Coconut Chip Cookies

Preparation Time: 10 minutes

Cooking Time: 15 minutes

Servings: 4

Ingredients :

- 1 cup almond flour
- ½ cup cacao nibs
- ½ cup coconut flakes, unsweetened
- 1/3 cup erythritol
- ½ cup almond butter
- ¼ cup nut butter, melted
- ¼ cup almond milk
- Stevia, to taste
- ¼ teaspoon sea salt

Directions:

1. Preheat your oven to 350 degrees F.

2. Layer a cookie sheet with parchment paper.

3. Add and then combine all the dry Ingredients in a glass bowl.

4. Whisk in butter, almond milk, vanilla essence, stevia, and almond butter.

5. Beat well then stir in dry mixture. Mix well.

6. Spoon out a tablespoon of cookie dough on the cookie sheet.

7. Add more dough to make as many as 16 cookies.

8. Flatten each cookie using your fingers.

9. Bake for 25 minutes until golden brown.

10. Let them sit for 15 minutes.

11. Serve.

Nutrition:

Calories 192

Total Fat 17.44 g

Saturated Fat 11.5 g

Cholesterol 125 mg

Total Carbs 2.2 g

Sugar 1.4 g

Fiber 2.1 g

Sodium 135 mg

Protein 4.7 g

Peanut Butter Bars

Preparation Time: 10 minutes

Cooking Time: 10 minutes

Servings: 6

Ingredients :

• 3/4 cup almond flour

• 2 oz. almond butter

• 1/4 cup Swerve

• 1/2 cup peanut butter

• 1/2 teaspoon vanilla

Directions:

1. Combine all the Ingredients for bars.

2. Transfer this mixture to 6-inch small pan. Press it firmly.

3. Refrigerate for 30 minutes.

4. Slice and serve.

Nutrition:

Calories 214

Total Fat 19 g

Saturated Fat 5.8 g

Cholesterol 15 mg

Total Carbs 6.5 g

Sugar 1.9 g

Fiber 2.1 g

Sodium 123 mg

Protein 6.5 g

Zucchini Bread Pancakes

Preparation Time: 15 minutes

Cooking Time: 35 minutes

Servings: 3

Ingredients :

• Grapeseed oil, 1 tbsp.

• Chopped walnuts, .5 c

• Walnut milk, 2 c

• Shredded zucchini, 1 c

• Mashed burro banana, .25 c

• Date sugar, 2 tbsp.

• Kamut flour or spelt, 2 c

Directions:

1. Place the date sugar and flour into a bowl. Whisk together.

2. Add in the mashed banana and walnut milk. Stir until combined. Remember to scrape the bowl to get all the dry mixture. Add in walnuts and zucchini. Stir well until combined.

3. Place the grapeseed oil onto a griddle and warm.

4. Pour .25 cup batter on the hot griddle. Leave it along until bubbles begin forming on to surface. Carefully turn over the pancake and cook another four minutes until cooked through.

5. Place the pancakes onto a serving plate and enjoy with some agave syrup.

Nutrition:

Calories: 246

Carbohydrates: 49.2 g

Fiber: 4.6 g

Protein: 7.8 g

Berry Sorbet

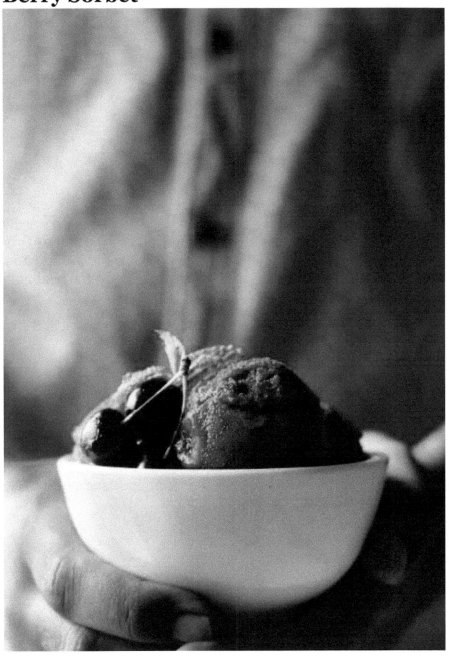

Preparation Time: 10 minutes

Cooking Time: 20 minutes

Servings: 6

Ingredients :

• Water, 2 c

• Blend strawberries, 2 c

• Spelt Flour, 1.5 tsp.

• Date sugar, .5 c

Directions:

1. Add the water into a large pot and let the water begin to warm. Add the flour and date sugar and stir until dissolved. Allow this mixture to start boiling and continue to cook for around ten minutes. It should have started to thicken. Take off the heat and set to the side to cool.

2. Once the syrup has cooled off, add in the strawberries, and stir well to combine.

3. Pour into a container that is freezer safe and put it into the freezer until frozen.

4. Take sorbet out of the freezer, cut into chunks, and put it either into a blender or a food processor. Hit the pulse button until the mixture is creamy.

5. Pour this into the same freezer-safe container and put it back into the freezer for four minutes.

Nutrition:

Calories: 99

Carbohydrates: 8 g

Quinoa Porridge

Preparation Time: 5 minutes

Cooking Time: 15 minutes

Servings: 04

Ingredients :

• Zest of one lime

• Coconut milk, .5 c

• Cloves, .5 tsp.

• Ground ginger, 1.5 tsp.

• Spring water, 2 c

• Quinoa, 1 c

• Grated apple, 1

Directions:

1. Cook the quinoa. Follow the instructions on the package. When the quinoa has been cooked, drain well. Place it back into the pot and stir in spices.

2. Add coconut milk and stir well to combine.

3. Grate the apple now and stir well.

4. Divide equally into bowls and add the lime zest on top. Sprinkle with nuts and seeds of choice.

Nutrition:

Calories: 180

Fat: 3 g

Carbohydrates: 40 g

Protein: 10 g

Apple Quinoa

Preparation Time: 15 minutes

Cooking Time: 30 minutes

Servings: 04

Ingredients :

• Coconut oil, 1 tbsp.

• Ginger

• Key lime .5

• Apple, 1

• Quinoa, .5 c

• Optional toppings

• Seeds

• Nuts

• Berries

Directions:

1. Fix the quinoa according to the instructions on the package. When you are getting close to the end of the Cooking time, grate in the apple and cook for 30 seconds.

2. Zest the lime into the quinoa and squeeze the juice in. Stir in the coconut oil.

3. Divide evenly into bowls and sprinkle with some ginger.

4. You can add in some berries, nuts, and seeds right before you eat.

Nutrition:

Calories: 146

Fiber: 2.3 g

Fat: 8.3 g

Kamut Porridge

Preparation Time: 10 minutes

Cooking Time: 25 minutes

Servings: 04

Ingredients :

• Agave syrup, 4 tbsp.

• Coconut oil, 1 tbsp.

• Sea salt, .5 tsp.

• Coconut milk, 3.75 c

• Kamut berries, 1 c

• Optional toppings

• Berries

• Coconut chips

• Ground nutmeg

• Ground cloves

Directions:

1. You need to "crack" the Kamut berries. You can try this by placing the berries into a food processor and pulsing until you have **1.** 25 cups of Kamut.

2. Place the cracked Kamut in a pot with salt and coconut milk. Give it a good stir in order to combine everything. Allow this mixture to come to a full rolling boil and then turn the heat down until the mixture is simmering. Stir every now and then until the Kamut has thickened to your likeness. This normally takes about ten minutes.

3. Take off heat, stir in agave syrup and coconut oil.

4. Garnish with toppings of choice and enjoy.

Nutrition:

Calories: 114

Protein: 5 g

Carbohydrates: 24g

Fiber: 4 g

Hot Kamut With Peaches, Walnuts, And Coconut

Preparation Time: 10 minutes

Cooking Time: 35 minutes

Servings: 04

Ingredients :

• Toasted coconut, 4 tbsp.

• Toasted and chopped walnuts, .5 c

• Chopped dried peaches, 8

• Coconut milk, 3 c

• Kamut cereal, 1 c

Directions:

1. Mix the coconut milk into a saucepan and allow it to warm up. When it begins simmering, add in the Kamut. Let this cook about 15 minutes, while stirring every now and then.

2. When done, divide evenly into bowls and top with the toasted coconut, walnuts, and peaches.

3. You could even go one more and add some fresh berries.

Nutrition:

Calories: 156

Protein: 5.8 g

Carbohydrates: 25 g

Fiber: 6 g

Overnight "Oats"

Preparation Time: 5 minutes

Cooking Time: 0 minutes

Servings: 04

Ingredients :

- Berry of choice, .5 c

- Walnut butter, .5 tbsp.

- Burro banana, .5

- Ginger, .5 tsp.

- Coconut milk, .5 c

- Hemp seeds, .5 c

Directions:

1. Put the hemp seeds, salt, and coconut milk into a glass jar. Mix well.

2. Place the lid on the jar then put in the refrigerator to sit overnight.

3. The next morning, add the ginger, berries, and banana. Stir well and enjoy.

Nutrition:

Calories: 139

Fat: 4.1 g

Protein: 9 g

Sugar: 7 g

Brazil Nut Cheese

Preparation Time: 20 minutes

Cooking Time: 0 minutes

Servings: 04

Ingredients :

• Grapeseed oil, 2 tsp.

• Water, 1.5 c

• Hemp milk, 1.5 c

• Cayenne, .5 tsp.

• Onion powder, 1 tsp.

• Juice of .5 lime

• Sea salt, 2 tsp.

• Brazil nuts, 1 lb.

• Onion powder, 1 tsp.

Directions:

1. You will need to start process by soaking the Brazil nuts in some water. You just put the nuts into a bowl and make sure the water covers them. Soak no less than 20 minutes or overnight. Overnight would be best.

2. Now you need to put everything except water into a food processor or blender.

3. Add just .5 cups water and blend for two minutes

4. Continue adding .5 cup water and blending until you have the consistency you want.

5. Scrape into an airtight container and enjoy.

Nutrition:

Calories: 187

Protein: 4.1 g

Fat: 19 g

Carbs: 3.3 g

Fiber: 2.1 g

Baked Stuffed Pears

Preparation Time: 15 minutes

Cooking Time: 35 minutes

Servings: 04

Ingredients :

• Agave syrup, 4 tbsp.

• Cloves, .25 tsp.

• Chopped walnuts, 4 tbsp.

• Currants, 1 c

• Pears, 4

Directions:

1. Make sure your oven has been warmed to 375

2. Slice the pears in two lengthwise and remove the core. To get the pear to lay flat, you can slice a small piece off the back side.

3. Place the agave syrup, currants, walnuts, and cloves in a small bowl and mix well. Set this to the side to be used later.

4. Put the pears on a cookie sheet that has parchment paper on it. Make sure the cored sides are facing up. Sprinkle each pear half with about .5 tablespoon of the chopped walnut mixture.

5. Place into the oven and cook for 25 to 30 minutes. Pears should be tender.

Nutrition:

Calories: 103.9

Fiber: 3.1 g

Carbohydrates: 22 g

Butternut Squash Pie

Preparation Time: 25 minutes

Cooking Time: 35 minutes

Servings: 04

Ingredients :

- For the Crust
- Cold water
- Agave, splash
- Sea salt, pinch
- Grapeseed oil, .5 c
- Coconut flour, .5 c
- Spelt Flour, 1 c
- For the Filling
- Butternut squash, peeled, chopped
- Water
- Allspice, to taste
- Agave syrup, to taste
- Hemp milk, 1 c
- Sea moss, 4 tbsp.

Directions:

1. You will need to warm your oven to 350.

2. For the Crust

3. Place the grapeseed oil and water into the refrigerator to get it cold. This will take about 10 minutes.

4. Place all Ingredients into a large bowl. Now you need to add in the cold water a little bit in small amounts until a dough forms. Place this onto a surface that has been sprinkled with some coconut flour. Knead for a few minutes and roll the dough as thin as you can get it. Carefully, pick it up and place it inside a pie plate.

5. Place the butternut squash into a Dutch oven and pour in enough water to cover. Bring this to a full rolling boil. Let this cook until the squash has become soft.

6. Completely drain and place into bowl. Using a potato masher, mash the squash. Add in some allspice and agave to taste. Add in the sea moss and hemp milk. Using a hand mixer, blend well. Pour into the pie crust.

7. Place into an oven and bake for about 30 minutes.

Nutrition:

Calories: 245

Carbohydrates: 50 g

Fat: 10 g

Coconut Chia Cream Pot

Preparation Time: 5 minutes

Cooking Time: 5 minutes

Servings: 04

Ingredients :

• Date, one (1)

• Coconut milk (organic), one (1) cup

• Coconut yogurt, one (1) cup

• Vanilla extract, ½ teaspoon

• Chia seeds, ¼ cup

• Sesame seeds, one (1) teaspoon

• Flaxseed (ground), one (1) tablespoon or flax meal, one (1) tablespoon

• Toppings:

• Fig, one (1)

• Blueberries, one(1) handful

• Mixed nuts (brazil nuts, almonds, pistachios, macadamia, etc.)

• Cinnamon (ground), one teaspoon

Directions:

1. First, blend the date with coconut milk (the idea is to sweeten the coconut milk).

2. Get a mixing bowl and add the coconut milk with the vanilla, sesame seeds, chia seeds, and flax meal.

3. Refrigerate for between twenty to thirty minutes or wait till the chia expands.

4. To serve, pour a layer of coconut yogurt in a small glass, then add the chia mix, followed by pouring another layer of the coconut yogurt.

5. It's alkaline, creamy and delicious.

Nutrition:

Calories: 310

Carbohydrates: 39 g

Protein: 4 g

Fiber: 8.1 g

Chocolate Avocado Mousse

Preparation Time: 10 minutes

Cooking Time: 5 minutes

Servings: 04

Ingredients :

• Coconut water, Servings cup

• Avocado, ½ hass

• Raw cacao, 2 teaspoons

• Vanilla, 1 teaspoon

• Dates, three (3)

• Sea salt, one (1) teaspoon

• Dark chocolate shavings

Directions:

1. Blend all Ingredients.

2. Blast until it becomes thick and smooth, as you wish.

3. Put in a fridge and allow it to get firm.

Nutrition:

Calories: 181.8

Fat: 151 g

Protein: 12 g

Chia Vanilla Coconut Pudding

Preparation Time: 5 minutes

Cooking Time: 5 minutes

Servings: 2

Ingredients :

• Coconut oil, 2 tablespoons

• Raw cashew, ½ cup

• Coconut water, ½ cup

• Cinnamon, 1 teaspoon

• Dates (pitted), 3

• Vanilla, 2 teaspoons

• Coconut flakes (unsweetened), 1 teaspoon

• Salt (Himalayan or Celtic Grey)

• Chia seeds, 6 tablespoons

• Cinnamon or pomegranate seeds for garnish (optional)

Directions:

1. Get a blender, add all the Ingredients (minus the pomegranate and chia seeds), and blend for about forty to sixty seconds.

2. Reduce the blender speed to the lowest and add the chia seeds.

3. Pour the content into an airtight container and put in a refrigerator for 25 minutes.

4. To serve, you can garnish with the cinnamon powder of pomegranate seeds.

Nutrition:

Calories: 201

Fat: 10 g

Sodium: 32.8 mg

Sweet Tahini Dip With Ginger Cinnamon Fruit

Preparation Time: 10 minutes

Cooking Time: 5 minutes

Servings: 2

Ingredients :

• Cinnamon, one (1) teaspoon

• Green apple, one (1)

• Pear, one (1)

• Fresh ginger, two (2) – three (3)

• Celtic sea salt, one (1) teaspoon

• Ingredient for sweet Tahini

• Almond butter (raw), three (3) teaspoons

• Tahini (one big scoop), three (3) teaspoons

• Coconut oil, two (2) teaspoons

• Cayenne (optional), ¼ teaspoons

• Wheat-free tamari, two (2) teaspoons

• Liquid coconut nectar, one (1) teaspoon

Directions:

1. Get a clean mixing bowl.

2. Grate the ginger, add cinnamon, sea salt and mix together in the bowl.

3. Dice apple and pear into little cubes, turn into the bowl and mix.

4. Get a mixing bowl and mix all the Ingredients.

5. Then add the Sprinkle the Sweet Tahini Dip all over the Ginger Cinnamon Fruit.

6. Serve.

Nutrition:

Calories: 109

Fat: 10.8 g

Sodium: 258 mg

Coconut Butter And Chopped Berries With Mint

Preparation Time: 5 minutes

Cooking Time: 5 minutes

Servings: 04

Ingredients :

• Chopped mint, one (1) tablespoon

• Coconut butter (melted), two (2) tablespoons

• Mixed berries (strawberries, blueberries, and raspberries)

Directions:

1. Get a small bowl and add the berries.

2. Drizzle the melted coconut butter and sprinkle the mint.

3. Serve.

Nutrition:

Calories: 159

Fat: 12 g

Carbohydrates: 18 g

Alkaline Raw Pumpkin Pie

Preparation Time: 5 minutes

Cooking Time: 5 minutes

Servings: 04

Ingredients :

Ingredients for Pie Crust

• Cinnamon, one (1) teaspoon

• Dates/Turkish apricots, one (1) cup

• Raw almonds, one (1) cup

• Coconut flakes (unsweetened), one (1) cup

Ingredients for Pie Filling

• Dates, six (6)

• Cinnamon, ½ teaspoon

• Nutmeg, ½ teaspoon

• Pecans (soaked overnight), one (1) cup

• Organic pumpkin Blends (12 oz.), 1 ¼ cup

• Nutmeg, ½ teaspoon

• Sea salt (Himalayan or Celtic Sea Salt), ¼ teaspoon

• Vanilla, 1 teaspoon

• Gluten-free tamari

Directions:

Directions for pie crust

1. Get a food processor and blend all the pie crust Ingredients at the same time.

2. Make sure the mixture turns oily and sticky before you stop mixing.

3. Put the mixture in a pie pan and mold against the sides and floor, to make it stick properly.

Directions for the pie filling

1. Mix Ingredients together in a blender.

2. Add the mixture to fill in the pie crust.

3. Pour some cinnamon on top.

4. Then refrigerate till it's cold.

5. Then mold.

Nutrition:

Calories 135

Calories from Fat 41.4

Total Fat 4.6 g

Cholesterol 11.3 mg

Strawberry Sorbet

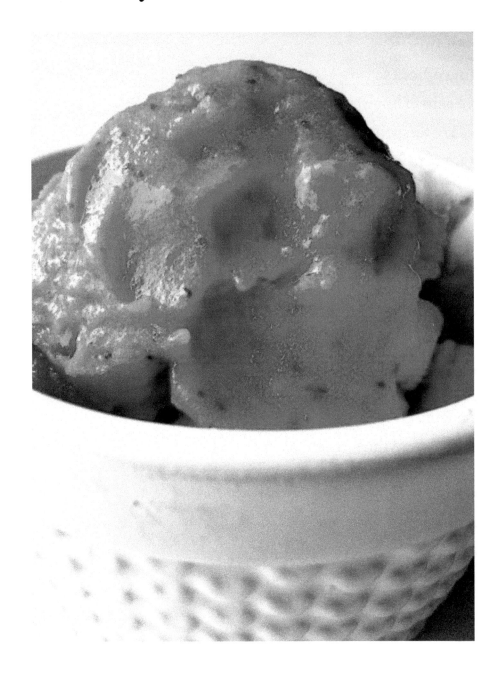

Preparation Time: 5 minutes

Cooking Time: 40 minutes

Servings: 4

Ingredients :

• 2 cups of Strawberries*

• 1 1/2 teaspoons of Spelt Flour

• 1/2 cup of Date Sugar

• 2 cups of Spring Water

Directions:

• Add Date Sugar, Spring Water, and Spelt Flour to a medium pot and boil on low heat for about ten minutes. Mixture should thicken, like syrup.

• Remove the pot from the heat and allow it to cool.

• After cooling, add Blend Strawberry and mix gently.

• Put mixture in a container and freeze.

• Cut it into pieces, put the sorbet into a processor and blend until smooth.

• Put everything back in the container and leave in the refrigerator for at least 35 minutes.

• Serve and enjoy your Strawberry Sorbet!

Nutrition:

Calories: 198

Carbohydrates: 28 g

Blueberry Cupcakes

Preparation Time: 5 minutes

Cooking Time: 10 minutes

Servings: 3

Ingredients :

• 1/2 cup of Blueberries

• 3/4 cup of Teff Flour

• 3/4 cup of Spelt Flour

• 1/3 cup of Agave Syrup

• 1/2 teaspoon of Pure Sea Salt

• 1 cup of Coconut Milk

• 1/4 cup of Sea Moss Gel (optional, check information)

• Grape Seed Oil

Directions:

1. Preheat your oven to 365 degrees Fahrenheit.

2. Grease or line 6 standard muffin cups.

3. Add Teff, Spelt flour, Pure Sea Salt, Coconut Milk, Sea Moss Gel, and Agave Syrup to a large bowl. Mix them together.

4. Add Blueberries to the mixture and mix well.

5. Divide muffin batter among the 6 muffin cups.

6. Bake for 30 minutes until golden brown.

7. Serve and enjoy your Blueberry Muffins!

Nutrition:

Calories: 65

Fat: 0.7 g

Carbohydrates: 12 g

Protein: 1.4 g

Fiber: 5 g

Banana Strawberry Ice Cream

Preparation Time: 5 minutes

Cooking Time: 0 minutes

Servings: 5

Ingredients :

- 1 cup of Strawberry*
- 5 quartered Baby Bananas*
- 1/2 Avocado, chopped
- 1 tablespoon of Agave Syrup
- 1/4 cup of Homemade Walnut Milk

Directions:

1. Mix **Ingredients** into the blender and blend them well.

2. Taste. If it is too thick, add extra Milk or Agave Syrup if you want it sweeter.

3. Put in a container with a lid and allow to freeze for at least 35 minutes.

4. Serve it and enjoy your Banana Strawberry Ice Cream!

Nutrition:

Calories: 200

Fat: 0.5 g

Carbohydrates: 44 g

Homemade Whipped Cream

Preparation Time: 5 minutes

Cooking Time: 10 Minutes

Servings: 1 Cup

Ingredients :

• 1 cup of Aquafaba

• 1/4 cup of Agave Syrup

Directions:

1. Add Agave Syrup and Aquafaba into a bowl.

2. Mix at high speed around 5 minutes with a stand mixer or 10 to 15 minutes with a hand mixer.

3. Serve and enjoy your Homemade Whipped Cream!

Nutrition:

Calories: 21

Fat: 0g

Sodium: 0.3g

Carbohydrates: 5.3g

Fiber: 0g

Sugars: 4.7g

Protein: 0g

"Chocolate" Pudding

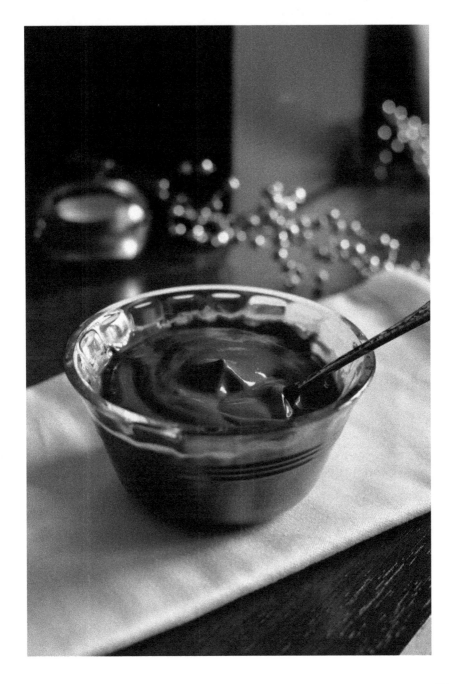

Preparation Time: 5 minutes

Cooking Time: 20 Minutes

Servings: 4

Ingredients :

• 1 to 2 cups of Black Sapote

• 1/4 cup of Agave Syrup

• 1/2 cup of soaked Brazil Nuts

• 1 tablespoon of Hemp Seeds

• 1/2 cup of Spring Water

Directions:

1. Cut 1 to 2 cups of Black Sapote in half.

2. Remove all seeds. You should have 1 full cup of de-seeded fruit.

3. Mix all Ingredients into a blender and blend until smooth.

4. Serve and enjoy your "Chocolate" Pudding!

Nutrition:

Calories: 134

Fat: 0.5 g

Carbohydrates: 15 g

Protein: 2.5 g

Fiber: 10 g

Banana Nut Muffins

Preparation Time: 5 minutes

Cooking Time: 30 minutes

Servings: 6

Ingredients

Dry Ingredients:

• 1 1/2 cups of Spell or Teff Flour

• 1/2 teaspoon of Pure Sea Salt

• 3/4 cup of Date Syrup

Wet Ingredients:

• 2 medium Blendd Burro Bananas

• ¼ cup of Grape Seed Oil

• ¾ cup of Homemade Walnut Milk (see recipe)*

• 1 tablespoon of Key Lime Juice

Filling Ingredients:

• ½ cup of chopped Walnuts (plus extra for decorating)

• 1 chopped Burro Banana

Directions:

1. Preheat your oven to 400 degrees Fahrenheit.

2. Take a muffin tray and grease 12 cups or line with cupcake liners.

3. Put all dry Ingredients in a large bowl and mix them thoroughly.

4. Add all wet Ingredients to a separate, smaller bowl and mix well with Blendd Bananas.

5. Mix Ingredients from the two bowls in one large container. Be careful not to over mix.

6. Add the filling Ingredients and fold in gently.

7. Pour muffin batter into the 12 prepared muffin cups and garnish with a couple Walnuts.

8. Bake it for 22 to 26 minutes until golden brown.

9. Allow to cool for 10 minutes.

10. Serve and enjoy your Banana Nut Muffins!

Nutrition:

Calories: 150

Fat: 10 g

Carbohydrates: 30 g

Protein: 2.4 g

Fiber: 2 g

Blackberry Jam

Preparation Time: 5 minutes

Cooking Time: 30 Minutes

Servings: 1 Cup

Ingredients :

• 3/4 cup of Blackberries

• 1 tablespoon of Key Lime Juice

• 3 tablespoons of Agave Syrup

• ¼ cup of Sea Moss Gel + extra 2 tablespoons (check information)

Directions:

1. Put rinsed Blackberries into a medium pot and cook on medium heat.

2. Stir Blackberries until liquid appears.

3. Once berries soften, use your immersion blender to chop up any large pieces. If you don't have a blender put the mixture in a food processor, mix it well, then return to the pot.

4. Add Sea Moss Gel, Key Lime Juice and Agave Syrup to the blended mixture. Boil on medium heat and stir well until it becomes thick.

5. Remove from the heat and leave it to cool for 10 minutes.

6. Serve it with bread pieces or the Flatbread (see recipe).

7. Enjoy your Blackberry Jam!

Nutrition:

Calories: 43

Fat: 0.5 g

Carbohydrates: 13 g

Blackberry Bars

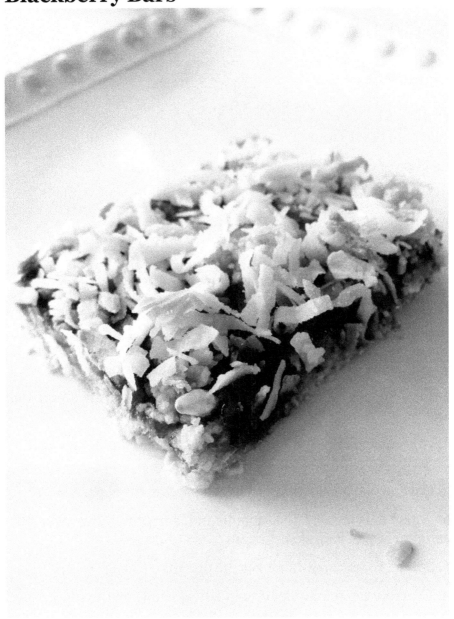

Preparation Time: 5 minutes

Cooking Time: 20 Minutes

Servings: 4

Ingredients :

• 3 Burro Bananas or 4 Baby Bananas

• 1 cup of Spelt Flour

• 2 cups of Quinoa Flakes

• 1/4 cup of Agave Syrup

• 1/4 teaspoon of Pure Sea Salt

• 1/2 cup of Grape Seed Oil

• 1 cup of prepared Blackberry Jam

Directions:

1. Preheat your oven to 350 degrees Fahrenheit.

2. Remove skin of Bananas and mash with a fork in a large bowl.

3. Combine Agave Syrup and Grape Seed Oil with the Blend and mix well.

4. Add Spelt Flour and Quinoa Flakes. Knead the dough until it becomes sticky to your fingers.

5. Cover a 9x9-inch baking pan with parchment paper.

6. Take Servings of the dough and smooth it out over the parchment pan with your fingers.

7. Spread Blackberry Jam over the dough.

8. Crumble the remainder dough and sprinkle on the top.

9. Bake for 20 minutes.

10. Remove from the oven and let it cool for at 10 to 15 minutes.

11. Cut into small pieces.

12. Serve and enjoy your Blackberry Bars!

Nutrition:

Calories: 43

Fat: 0.5 g

Carbohydrates: 10 g

Protein: 1.4 g

Fiber: 5 g

Detox Berry Smoothie

Preparation Time: 15 minutes

Cooking Time: 0

Servings: 1

Ingredients :

• Spring water

• 1/4 avocado, pitted

• One medium burro banana

• One Seville orange

• Two cups of fresh lettuce

• One tablespoon of hemp seeds

• One cup of berries (blueberries or an aggregate of blueberries, strawberries, and raspberries)

Directions:

1. Add the spring water to your blender.

2. Put the fruits and vegies right inside the blender.

3. Blend all Ingredients till smooth.

Nutrition:

Calories: 202.4

Fat: 4.5g

Carbohydrates: 32.9g

Protein: 13.3g

Spinach And Sesame Crackers

Preparation Time: 5 minutes

Cooking Time: 15 minutes

Servings: 4

Ingredients :

- 2 tablespoons white sesame seeds

- 1 cup fresh spinach, washed

- 1 Servings cups all-purpose flour

- 1/2 cup water

- 1/2 teaspoon baking powder

- 1 teaspoon olive oil

- 1 teaspoon salt

Directions:

1. Transfer the spinach to a blender with a half cup water and blend until smooth.

2. Add 2 tablespoons white sesame seeds, ½ teaspoon baking powder, 1 Servings cups all-purpose flour, and 1 teaspoon salt to a bowl and stir well until combined. Add in 1 teaspoon olive oil and spinach water. Mix again and knead by using your hands until you obtain a smooth dough.

3. If the made dough is too gluey, then add more flour.

4. Using your parchment paper lightly roll out the dough as thin as possible. Cut into squares with a pizza cutter.

5. Bake into a preheated oven at 400°, for about 15to 20 minutes. Once done, let cool and then serve.

Nutrition:

223 calories

3g fat

41g total carbohydrates

6g protein

Mini Nacho Pizzas

Preparation Time: 5 minutes

Cooking Time: 10 minutes

Servings: 4

Ingredients :

- 1/4 cup refried beans, vegan
- 2 tablespoons tomato, diced
- 2 English muffins, split in half
- 1/4 cup onion, sliced
- 1/3 cup vegan cheese, shredded
- 1 small jalapeno, sliced
- 1/3 cup roasted tomato salsa
- 1/2 avocado, diced and tossed in lemon juice

Directions:

1. Add the refried beans/salsa onto the muffin bread. Sprinkle with shredded vegan cheese followed by the veggie toppings.

2. Transfer to a baking sheet and place in a preheated oven at 350 to 400 F on a top rack.

3. Put into the oven for 10 minutes and then broil for 2minutes, so that the top becomes bubbly.

4. Take out from the oven and let them cool at room temperature.

5. Top with avocado. Enjoy!

Nutrition:

133 calories

4.2g fat

719g total carbohydrates

6g protein

Pizza Sticks

Preparation Time: 10 minutes

Cooking Time: 30 minutes

Servings: 16 sticks

Ingredients :

• 5 tablespoons tomato sauce

• Few pinches of dried basil

• 1 block extra firm tofu

• 2 tablespoon + 2 teaspoon Nutritional yeast

Directions:

1. Cape the tofu in a paper tissue and put a cutting board on top, place something heavy on top and drain for about 10 to 15 minutes.

2. In the meantime, line your baking sheet with parchment paper. Cut the tofu into 16 equal pieces and place them on a baking sheet.

3. Spread each pizza stick with a teaspoon of marinara sauce.

4. Sprinkle each stick with half teaspoon of yeast, followed by basil on top.

5. Bake into a preheated oven at 425 F for about 28 to 30 minutes. Serve and enjoy!

Nutrition:

33 calories

1.7g fat

2g total carbs

3g protein

Raw Broccoli Poppers

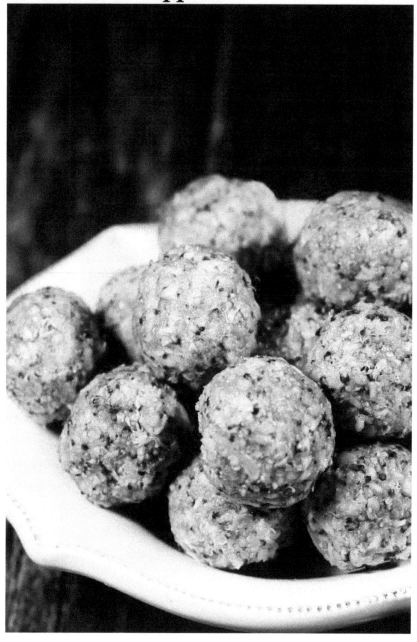

Preparation Time: 2 minutes

Cooking Time: 8 minutes

Servings: 4

Ingredients :

• 1/8 cup water

• 1/8 teaspoon fine sea salt

• 4 cups broccoli florets, washed and cut into 1-inch pieces

• 1/4 teaspoon turmeric powder

• 1 cup unsalted cashews, soaked for at least 30 minutes and drained

• 1/4 teaspoon onion powder

• 1 red bell pepper, seeded and

• 2 heaping tablespoons Nutritional

• 2 tablespoons lemon juice

Directions:

1. Transfer the drained cashews to a high speed blender and pulse for about 30 seconds. Add in the chopped pepper and pulse again for 30seconds.

2. Add some 2 tablespoons lemon juice, 1/8 cup water, 2heaping tablespoons Nutritional yeast, ¼ teaspoon onion powder, 1/8 teaspoon fine sea salt, and 1/4 teaspoon turmeric powder. Pulse for about 45 seconds until smooth.

3. Handover the broccoli into a bowl and add in chopped cheesy cashew mixture. Toss well until coated.

4. Transfer the pieces of broccoli to the trays of a yeast dehydrator.

5. Follow the dehydrator's instructions and dehydrate for about 8 minutes at 125 F or until crunchy.

Nutrition:

408 calories

32g fat

22g total carbohydrates

15g protein

Blueberry Cauliflower

Preparation Time: 2 minutes

Cooking Time: 5 minutes

Servings: 1

Ingredients :

• ¼ cup frozen strawberries

• 2 teaspoons maple syrup

• ¾ cup unsweetened cashew milk

• 1 teaspoon vanilla extract

• ½ cup plain cashew yogurt

• 5 tablespoons powdered peanut butter

• ¾ cup frozen wild blueberries

• ½ cup cauliflower florets, coarsely chopped

Directions:

1. Add all the smoothie Ingredients to a high speed blender.

2. Blitz to combine until smooth.

3. Pour into a chilled glass and serve.

Nutrition:

340 calories

11g fat

48g total carbohydrates

16g protein

Candied Ginger

Preparation Time: 10 minutes

Cooking Time: 40 minutes

Servings: 3 to 5

Ingredients :

• 2 1/2 cups salted pistachios, shelled

• 1 1/4 teaspoons powdered ginger

• 3 tablespoons pure maple syrup

Directions:

1. Add 1 1/4 teaspoons powdered ginger to a bowl with pistachios. Stir well until combined. There

2. should be no lumps.

3. Drizzle with 3 tablespoons of maple syrup and stir well.

4. Transfer to a baking sheet lined with parchment paper and spread evenly.

5. Cook into a preheated oven at 275 F for about 20 minutes.

6. Take out from oven, stir, and cook for further 10 to 15 minutes.

7. Let it cool for about few minutes until crispy. Enjoy!

Nutrition:

378 calories

27.6g fat

26g total carbohydrates

13g protein

Chia Crackers

Preparation Time: 20 minutes

Cooking Time: 10 minutes

Servings: 24-26 crackers

Ingredients :

- 1/2 cup pecans, chopped
- 1/2 cup chia seeds
- 1/2 teaspoon cayenne pepper
- 1 cup water
- 1/4 cup Nutritional yeast
- 1/2 cup pumpkin seeds
- 1/4 cup ground flax
- Salt and pepper, to taste

Directions:

1. Mix around 1/2 cup chia seeds and 1 cup water. Keep it aside.

2. Take another bowl and combine all the remaining Ingredients. Combine well and stir in the chia water mixture until you obtained dough.

3. Transfer the dough onto a baking sheet and rollout (¼" thick).

4. Transfer into a preheated oven at 325°F and bake for about 30 minutes.

5. Take out from the oven, flip over the dough, and cut it into desired cracker shape/squares.

6. Spread and back again for further 30 minutes, or until crispy and browned.

7. Once done, take out from oven and let them cool at room temperature. Enjoy!

Nutrition:

41 calories

3. 1g fat

2g total carbohydrates

2g protein

Orange- Spiced Pumpkin Hummus

Preparation Time: 2 minutes

Cooking Time: 5 minutes

Servings: 4 cups

Ingredients :

• 1 tablespoon maple syrup

• 1/2 teaspoon salt

• 1 can (16oz.) garbanzo beans,

• 1/8 teaspoon ginger or nutmeg

• 1 cup canned pumpkin Blend,

• 1/8 teaspoon cinnamon

• 1/4 cup tahini

• 1 tablespoon fresh orange juice

• Pinch of orange zest, for garnish

• 1 tablespoon apple cider vinegar

Directions:

1. Mix all the Ingredients to a food processor blender and blend until slightly chunky.

2. Serve right away and enjoy!

Nutrition:

291 calories

22.9g fat

15g total carbohydrates

12g protein

Cinnamon Maple Sweet Potato Bites

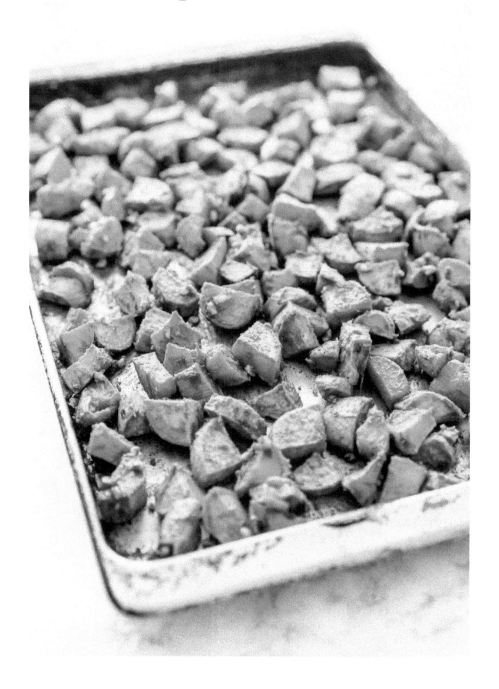

Preparation Time: 5 minutes

Cooking Time: 25 minutes

Servings: 3 to 4

Ingredients :

• ½ teaspoon corn-starch

• 1 teaspoon cinnamon

• 4 medium sweet potatoes, then peeled, and cut into bite-size cubes

• 2 to 3 tablespoons maple syrup

• 3 tablespoons butter, melted

Directions:

1. Transfer the potato cubes to a Ziploc bag and add in 3 tablespoons of melted butter. Seal and shake well until the potato cubes are coated with butter.

2. Add in the remaining Ingredients and shake again.

3. Transfer the potato cubes to a parchment-lined baking sheet. Cubes shouldn't be stacked on one another.

4. Sprinkle with cinnamon, if needed, and bake in a preheated oven at 425°F for about 25 to 30 minutes, stirring once during cooking.

5. Once done, take them out and stand at room temperature. Enjoy!

Nutrition:

436 calories

17.4g fat

71.8g total carbohydrates

4.1g protein

Cheesy Kale Chips

Preparation Time: 3 minutes

Cooking Time: 12 minutes

Servings: 4

Ingredients :

- 3 tablespoons Nutritional yeast
- 1 head curly kale, washed, ribs
- 3/4 teaspoon garlic powder
- 1 tablespoon olive oil
- 1 teaspoon onion powder
- Salt, to taste

Directions:

1. Line cookie sheets with parchment paper.

2. Drain the kale leaves and spread on a paper removed and leaves torn into chip-

3. towel. Then, kindly transfer the leaves to a bowl and sized pieces

4. add in 1 teaspoon onion powder, 3 tablespoons Nutritional yeast, 1 tablespoon olive oil, and 3/4

5. teaspoon garlic powder. Mix with your hands.

6. Spread the kale onto prepared cookie sheets. They shouldn't touch each other.

7. Bake into a preheated oven for about 350 F for about 10to 12 minutes.

8. Once crisp, take out from the oven, and sprinkle with a bit of salt. Serve and enjoy!

Nutrition:

71 calories

4g fat

5g total carbohydrates

4g protein

Lemon Roasted Bell Pepper

Preparation Time: 10 minutes

Cooking Time: 5 minutes

Servings: 4

Ingredients :

• 4 bell peppers

• 1 teaspoon olive oil

• 1 tablespoon mango juice

• 1/4 teaspoon garlic, minced

• 1 teaspoons oregano

• 1 pinch salt

• 1 pinch pepper

Directions:

1. Start heating the Air Fryer to 390 degrees F

2. Place some bell pepper in the Air fryer

3. Drizzle it with the olive oil and air fry for 5 minutes

4. Take a serving plate and transfer it

5. Take a small bowl and add garlic, oregano, mango juice, salt, and pepper

6. Mix them well and drizzle the mixture over the peppers

7. Serve and enjoy!

Nutrition:

Calories: 59 kcal

Carbohydrates: 6 g

Fat: 5 g

Protein: 4 g

Subtle Roasted Mushrooms

Preparation Time: 10 minutes

Cooking Time: 5 minutes

Servings: 4

Ingredients :

• 2 teaspoons mixed Sebi Friendly herbs

• 1 tablespoon olive oil

• 1/2 teaspoon garlic powder

• 2 pounds mushrooms

• 2 tablespoons date sugar

Directions:

1. Wash mushrooms and turn dry in a plate of mixed greens spinner

2. Quarter them and put in a safe spot

3. Put garlic, oil, and spices in the dish of your oar type air fryer

4. Warmth for 2 minutes

5. Stir it.

6. Add some mushrooms and cook 25 minutes

7. Then include vermouth and cook for 5 minutes more

8. Serve and enjoy!

Nutrition:

Calories: 94 kcal

Carbohydrates: 3 g

Fat: 8 g

Protein: 2 g.

Fancy Spelt Bread

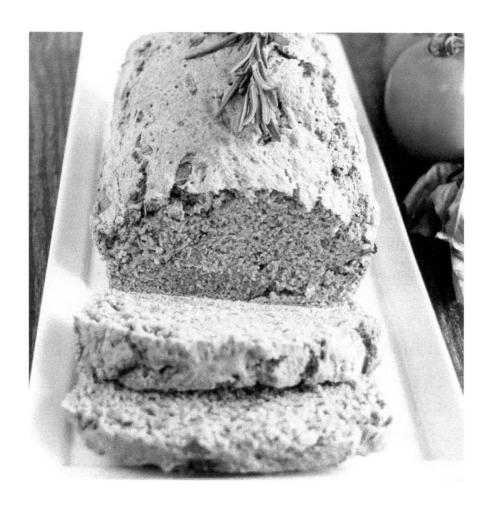

Preparation Time: 10 minutes

Cooking Time: 5 minutes

Servings: 4

Ingredients :

• 1 cup spring water

• 1/2 cup of coconut milk

• 3 tablespoons avocado oil

• 1 teaspoon baking soda

• 1 tablespoon agave nectar

• 4 and 1/2 cups spelt flour

• 1 and 1/2 teaspoon salt

Directions:

1. Pre-heat your Air Fryer to 355 degrees F

2. Take a big bowl and add baking soda, salt, flour whisk well

3. Add 3/4 cup of water, plus coconut milk, oil and mix well

4. Sprinkle your working surface with flour, add dough to the flour

5. Roll well

6. Knead for about three minutes, adding small amounts of flour until dough is a nice ball

7. Place parchment paper in your cooking basket

8. Lightly grease your pan and put the dough inside

9. Transfer into Air Fryer and bake for 30 minutes until done

10. Remove then insert a stick to check for doneness

11. If done already serve and enjoy, if not, let it cook for a few minutes more

Nutrition:

Calories: 203 kcal

Carbohydrates: 37 g

Fat: 4g

Protein: 7 g

Crispy Crunchy Hummus

Preparation Time: 10 minutes

Cooking Time: 10-15 minutes

Servings: 4

Ingredients :

- 1/2 a red onion
- 2 tablespoons fresh coriander
- 1/4 cup cherry tomatoes
- 1/2 a red bell pepper
- 1 tablespoon dulse flakes
- Juice of lime
- Salt to taste
- 3 tablespoons olive oil
- 2 tablespoons tahini
- 1 cup warm chickpeas

Directions:

1. Prepare your Air Fryer cooking basket

2. Add chickpeas to your cooking container and cook for 10-15 minutes, making a point to continue blending them every once in a while until they are altogether warmed

3. Add warmed chickpeas to a bowl and include tahini, salt, lime

4. Utilize a fork to pound chickpeas and fixings in a glue until smooth

5. Include hacked onion, cherry tomatoes, ringer pepper, dulse drops, and olive oil

6. Blend well until consolidated

7. Serve hummus with a couple of cuts of spelt bread

Nutrition:

Calories: 95 kcal

Carbohydrates: 5 g

Fat: 5 g

Protein: 5 g

Chick Pea And Kale Dish

Preparation Time: 10 minutes

Cooking Time: 25-30 minutes

Servings: 4

Ingredients :

- 2 cups chickpea flour
- 1/2 cup green bell pepper, diced
- 1/2 cup onions, minced
- 1 tablespoon oregano
- 1 tablespoon salt
- 1 teaspoon cayenne
- 4 cups spring water
- 2 tablespoons Grape Seed Oil

Directions:

1. Boil spring water in a large pot

2. Lower heat into medium and whisk in chickpea flour

3. Add some minced onions, diced green bell pepper, seasoning to the pot and cook for 10 minutes

4. Cover dish using a baking sheet, grease with oil

5. Pour batter into the sheet and spread with a spatula

6. Cover with another sheet

7. Transfer to a fridge and chill, for 20 minutes

8. Remove from freezer and cut batter into fry shapes

9. Preheat the Air Fryer, to 385 degrees F

10. Transfer fries into the cooking basket, lightly greased and cover with parchment

11. Bake for about 15 minutes, flip and bake for 10 minutes more until golden brown

12. Serve and enjoy!

Nutrition:

Calories: 271 kcal

Carbohydrates: 28 g

Fat: 15 g

Protein: 9 g

Zucchini Chips

Preparation Time: 10 minutes

Cooking Time: 12-15 minutes

Servings: 4

Ingredients :

• Salt as needed

• Grape seed oil as needed

• 6 zucchinis

Directions:

1. Into 330 F, pre heat the Air Fryer

2. Wash zucchini, slice zucchini into thin strips

3. Put slices in a bowl and add oil, salt, and toss

4. Spread over the cooking basket, fry for 12-15 minutes

5. Serve and enjoy!

Nutrition:

Calories: 92 kcal

Carbohydrates: 6 g

Fat: 7 g

Protein: 2 g

Classic Blueberry Spelt Muffins

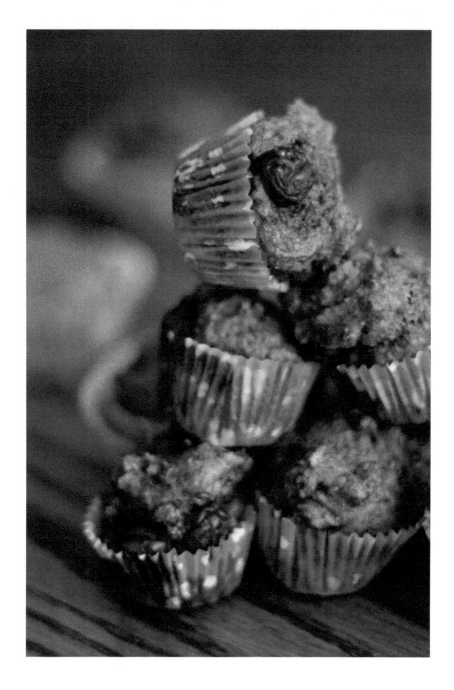

Preparation Time: 10 minutes

Cooking Time: 12-15 minutes

Servings: 4

Ingredients :

• 1/4 sea salt

• 1/3 cup maple syrup

• 1 teaspoon baking powder

• 1/2 cup sea moss

• 3/4 cup spelt flour

• 3/4 cup Kamut flour

• 1 cup hemp milk

• 1 cup blueberries

Directions:

1. Into 380 degrees F pre heat Air Fryer

2. Take your muffin tins and gently grease them

3. Take a bowl and add flour, syrup, salt, baking powder, seamless and mix well

4. Add milk and mix well

5. Fold in blueberries

6. Pour into muffin tins

7. Transfer to the cooking basket, bake for 20-25 minutes until nicely baked

8. Serve and enjoy!

Nutrition:

Calories: 217 kcal,

Carbohydrates: 32 g

Fat: 9 g

Protein: 4 g

Genuine Healthy Crackers

Preparation Time: 10 minutes

Cooking Time: 12-15 minutes

Servings: 4

Ingredients :

- 1/2 cup Rye flour

- 1 cup spelt flour

- 2 teaspoons sesame seed

- 1 teaspoon agave syrup

- 1 teaspoon salt

- 2 tablespoons grapeseed oil

- 3/4 cup spring water

Directions:

1. Into 330 degrees F, Preheat the Air Fryer

2. Take a medium bowl and add all Ingredients, mix well

3. Make dough ball

4. Prepare a place for rolling out the dough, cover with a piece of parchment

5. Lightly grease paper with grape seed oil, place dough

6. Roll out, dough with a rolling pin, add more flour if needed

7. Take a shape cutter and cut dough into squares

8. Place squares in Air Fryer cooking basket

9. Brush with more oil

10. Sprinkle salt

11. Bake for 10-15 minutes until golden

12. Let it cool, serve, and enjoy!

Nutrition:

Calories: 226 kcal

Carbohydrates: 41 g

Fat: 3 g

Protein: 11 g

Tortilla Chips

Preparation Time: 10 minutes

Cooking Time: 8-12 minutes

Servings: 4

Ingredients :

• 2 cups of spelt flour

• 1 teaspoon of salt

• 1/2 cup of spring water

• 1/3 cup of grapeseed oil

Directions:

1. Preheat your Air Fryer into 320 degrees F

2. Take the food processor then add salt, flour, and process well for 15 seconds

3. Gradually add grapeseed oil until mixed

4. Keep mixing until you have a nice dough

5. Formulate work surface and cover in a piece of parchment, sprinkle flour

6. Knead the dough for 1-2 minutes

7. Grease cooking basket with oil

8. Transfer dough on the cooking basket, brush oil and sprinkle salt

9. Cut dough into 8 triangles

10. Bake for about 8-12 minutes until golden brown

11. Serve and enjoy once done!

Nutrition:

Calories: 288 kcal

Carbohydrates: 18 g

Fat: 17 g

Protein: 16 g

Pumpkin Spice Crackers

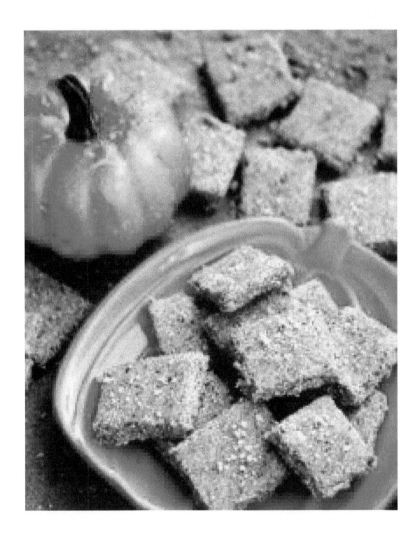

Preparation Time: 10 minutes

Cooking Time: 30 minutes

Servings: 06

Ingredients :

• 1⁄3 cup coconut flour

• 2 tablespoons pumpkin pie spice

• 3⁄4 cup sunflower seeds

• 3⁄4 cup flaxseed

• 1⁄3 cup sesame seeds

• 1 tablespoon ground psyllium husk powder

• 1 teaspoon sea salt

• 3 tablespoons coconut oil, melted

• 11⁄3 cups alkaline water

Directions:

1. Set your oven to 300 degrees F.

2. Combine all dry Ingredients in a bowl.

3. Add water and oil to the mixture and mix well.

4. Let the dough stay for 2 to 3 minutes.

5. Spread the dough evenly on a cookie sheet lined with parchment paper.

6. Bake for 30 minutes.

7. Reduce the oven heat to low and bake for another 30 minutes.

8. Crack the bread into bite-size pieces.

9. Serve

Nutrition:

Calories 248

Total Fat 15.7 g

Saturated Fat 2.7 g

Cholesterol 75 mg

Sodium 94 mg

Total Carbs 0.4 g

Fiber 0g

Sugar 0 g

Protein 24.9 g

Spicy Roasted Nuts

Preparation Time: 10 minutes

Cooking Time: 15 minutes

Servings: 4

Ingredients :

• 8 oz. pecans or almonds or walnuts

• 1 teaspoon sea salt

• 1 tablespoon olive oil or coconut oil

• 1 teaspoon ground cumin

• 1 teaspoon paprika powder or chili powder

Directions:

1. Add all the Ingredients to a skillet.

2. Roast the nuts until golden brown.

3. Serve and enjoy.

Nutrition:

Calories 287

Total Fat 29.5 g

Saturated Fat 3 g

Cholesterol 0 mg

Total Carbs 5.9 g

Sugar 1.4g

Fiber 4.3 g

Sodium 388 mg

Protein 4.2 g

Wheat Crackers

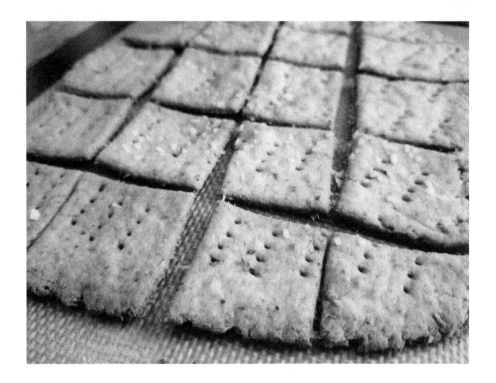

Preparation Time: 10 minutes

Cooking Time: 20 minutes

Servings: 4

Ingredients :

- 1 3/4 cups almond flour
- 1 1/2 cups coconut flour
- 3/4 teaspoon sea salt
- 1/3 cup vegetable oil
- 1 cup alkaline water
- Sea salt for sprinkling

Directions:

1. Set your oven to 350 degrees F.

2. Mix coconut flour, almond flour and salt in a bowl.

3. Stir in vegetable oil and water. Mix well until smooth.

4. Spread this dough on a floured surface into a thin sheet.

5. Cut small squares out of this sheet.

6. Arrange the dough squares on a baking sheet lined with parchment paper.

7. For about 20 minutes, bake until light golden in color.

8. Serve.

Nutrition:

Calories 64

Total Fat 9.2 g

Saturated Fat 2.4 g

Cholesterol 110 mg

Sodium 276 mg

Total Carbs 9.2 g

Fiber 0.9 g

Sugar 1.4 g

Protein 1.5 g

Potato Chips

Preparation Time: 10 minutes

Cooking Time: 20 minutes

Servings: 4

Ingredients :

• 1 tablespoon vegetable oil

• 1 potato, sliced paper thin

• Sea salt, to taste

Directions:

1. Toss potato with oil and sea salt.

2. Spread the slices in a baking dish in a single layer.

3. Cook in a microwave for 5 minutes until golden brown.

4. Serve.

Nutrition:

Calories 80

Total Fat 3.5 g

Saturated Fat 0.1 g

Cholesterol 320 mg

Sodium 350 mg

Total Carbs 11.6 g

Fiber 0.7 g

Sugar 0.7 g

Protein 1.2 g

Zucchini Pepper Chips

Preparation Time: 10 minutes

Cooking Time: 15 minutes

Servings: 04

Ingredients :

- 1 **Servings:** cups vegetable oil
- 1 teaspoon garlic powder
- 1 teaspoon onion powder
- 1/2 teaspoon black pepper
- 3 tablespoons crushed red pepper flakes
- 2 zucchinis, thinly sliced

Directions:

1. Mix oil with all the spices in a bowl.

2. Add zucchini slices and mix well.

3. Transfer the mixture to a Ziplock bag and seal it.

4. Refrigerate for 10 minutes.

5. Spread the zucchini slices on a greased baking sheet.

6. Bake for 15 minutes

7. Serve.

Nutrition:

Calories 172

Total Fat 11.1 g

Saturated Fat 5.8 g

Cholesterol 610 mg

Sodium 749 mg

Total Carbs 19.9 g

Fiber 0.2 g

Sugar 0.2 g

Protein 13.5 g

Kale Crisps

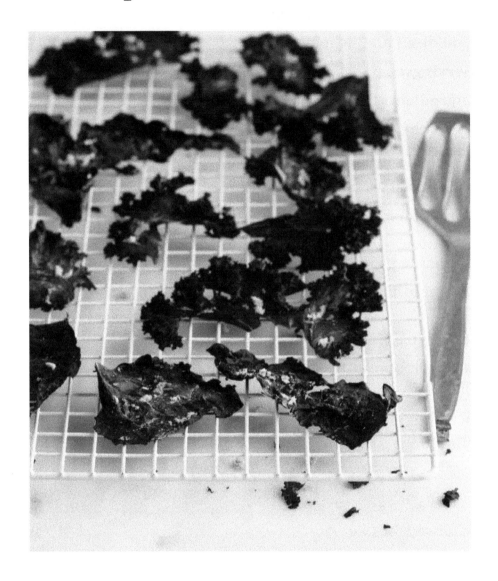

Preparation Time: 10 minutes

Cooking Time: 10 minutes

Servings: 04

Ingredients :

• 1 bunch kale, remove the stems, leaves torn into even pieces

• 1 tablespoon olive oil

• 1 teaspoon sea salt

Directions:

1. Set your oven to 350 degrees F. Layer a baking sheet with parchment paper.

2. Spread the kale leaves on a paper towel to absorb all the moisture.

3. Toss the leaves with sea salt, and olive oil.

4. Kindly spread them, on the baking sheet and bake for 10 minutes.

5. Serve.

Nutrition:

Calories 113

Total Fat 7.5 g

Saturated Fat 1.1 g

Cholesterol 20 mg

Sodium 97 mg

Total Carbs 1.4 g

Fiber 0 g

Sugar 0 g

Protein 1.1g

Lightning Source UK Ltd.
Milton Keynes UK
UKHW020656210521
384116UK00005B/101